ACUPRESSURE POINT FOR BEGINNERS

Unlocking Healing Paths, A Comprehensive Guide To Acupressure For Novices, Enhancing Wellness Naturally And Holistic Well-Being

LAMBERT FETTERMAN

DISCLAIMER

The content in this book is offered only for general informative purposes. While every effort has been taken to guarantee the content's accuracy and completeness, the author and publisher accept no responsibility for any mistakes or omissions, or for the results of using the information given herein. The methods, recommendations, and directions in this book are not guaranteed to be appropriate for every person, and readers should exercise caution and seek professional counsel if required before undertaking any of the projects or techniques detailed in this book.

Table of Contents

INTRODUCTION

Acupressure is an ancient therapeutic practice in which pressure is applied to certain spots on the body to improve energy flow and promote well-being. This section seeks to provide newcomers with a basic grasp of acupressure by delving into its fundamentals, historical origins, and differences from acupuncture.

Understanding Acupressure

Acupressure is based on the idea of vital energy, also known as Qi or Chi, flowing through the body's meridians or energy channels. Practitioners strive to balance and unblock the flow of energy by applying pressure to particular acupoints along these channels, treating a variety of physical and mental health conditions. This section will go over the essential concepts of acupressure and explain how it works to promote healing and good wellness.

The History And Origins Of Acupressure

Acupressure has a long history in traditional Chinese medicine, stretching back thousands of years. Understanding its historical background reveals the cultural and philosophical underpinnings of this activity. This section will look at the roots of acupressure, how it has evolved throughout time, and how it has been integrated into many holistic healing systems other than Chinese medicine.

How Acupressure Differs From Acupuncture

While acupressure and acupuncture have a theoretical underpinning, their applications vary. Acupuncture involves the insertion of small needles into particular acupoints, while acupressure depends on physical pressure without the necessity for skin penetration. This section will clarify the differences between the two modalities, assisting newcomers in understanding the unique qualities and benefits of acupressure.

Beginners may build the framework for their research of acupressure by getting a good knowledge of these initial topics. The next chapters will dig into the practical features, methods, and applications of acupressure, allowing people to include it in their wellness routines for a holistic approach to health and balance.

CHAPTER 1

Principles Of Acupressure

The Concept Of Qi And Meridians

Acupressure is based on the basic ideas of Qi (pronounced "chee") and meridians, which are rooted in ancient Chinese medicine. Qi is the essential life force energy that circulates throughout the body to maintain balance and wellness. Meridians are Qi-moving passageways that link numerous organs and bodily systems.

Recognizing the importance of Qi balance and free flow as important for well-being is the first step in understanding acupressure. When the Qi is blocked or imbalanced, it may cause bodily or emotional distress. By applying pressure to precise places along the meridians, acupressure seeks to restore equilibrium.

Yin And Yang In Acupressure

The ancient Chinese idea of Yin and Yang, which represents opposites and balance, is important in acupressure. In the context of acupressure, Yin represents stillness, darkness, and passivity, while Yang represents activity, light, and movement.

Acupressure attempts to balance the body's Yin and Yang energy. Each acupressure point correlates to either Yin or Yang and applying pressure to these points aids in the regulation of energy flow and the maintenance of balance.

The Five Elements Theory In Acupressure

Another fundamental principle in acupressure is the Five Elements Theory (Wood, Fire, Earth, Metal, and Water). Each element corresponds to certain organs, meridians, and emotions. Understanding this notion improves acupressure method accuracy.

• Wood: Wood indicates development and flexibility and is associated with the liver and gallbladder.

• Fire: Fire represents passion and change and is associated with the heart and small intestine.

• Earth: Earth governs the spleen and stomach and represents stability and nutrition.

• Metal: Metal represents clarity and strength and is associated with the lungs and big intestine.

• Water: Water denotes intelligence and adaptability and is associated with the kidneys and bladder.

Acupressure practitioners customize treatments to address particular imbalances connected to the organs and their associated elements by taking the Five Elements into account.

Understanding the concepts of Qi, Yin, and Yang, and the Five Elements sets the groundwork for efficient and comprehensive acupressure practice. These ideas help practitioners choose the right spots and procedures to boost the body's natural healing processes. Remember that each application of pressure is a step toward restoring balance and improving general well-being as you explore the realm of acupressure.

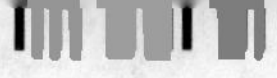

CHAPTER 2

Getting Started With Acupressure

Acupressure, a traditional Chinese medicine-based ancient therapeutic method, focuses on applying pressure to certain places on the body to encourage natural healing and relieve pain. Here's a full guide on getting started with acupressure:

Tools And Techniques

What You Need to Get Started Acupressure is typically applied with the fingers and hands. There are no complicated instruments necessary; however, some practitioners may use aids such as acupressure balls or rollers for certain methods. The goal is to perfect the application of pressure with your fingers.

Understanding Pressure Points

Understanding pressure points is fundamental to acupressure. These places are positioned along the meridians of the body, where vital energy (Qi) circulates. Each pressure point relates to a distinct organ or system of the body. It is essential to get acquainted with these topics and their related advantages.

Preparing For An Acupressure Session

Creating a suitable atmosphere is part of preparing for an acupressure session. Find a peaceful, comfortable place to rest where you won't be disturbed. Wear clothing that is loose and comfortable and offers easy access to the areas you plan to work on. Before beginning an acupressure session, take a few seconds to relax your thoughts and concentrate on your breathing.

This chapter lays the groundwork for novices to grasp the fundamentals of acupressure, from the fundamentals of pressure point identification to the bare minimum of instruments needed and the preliminary actions for a successful session.

CHAPTER 3

Exploring Key Acupressure Points

Acupressure is the application of pressure to certain places on the body to enhance natural healing powers and relieve pain. Understanding major acupressure points is essential for efficiently applying this ancient discipline.

Head And Neck Points

1. Governing Vessel (GV) 20 (Baihui): This vessel is located at the top of the head and is said to improve mental clarity and ease headaches.

2. Third Eye Point (GV 24.5 or Yintang): Located between the brows, it is associated with stress reduction and mind-calming.

3. Wind Pool (GB 20): This location, located near the base of the skull on each side of the spine, may assist in relieving neck strain and headaches.

Upper Body Points

1. Shoulder Well (GB 21): It is supposed to relieve shoulder and neck strain since it is located on the top of the shoulder.

2. Heart 7 (HT 7): This chakra is located on the wrist crease and is said to decrease anxiety and promote calm.

3. Large Intestine 4 (LI 4): Located on the back of the hand between the thumb and index finger, it is said to be beneficial for a variety of conditions, including headaches and sinus congestion.

Lower Body Points

1. Liver 3 (LV 3): It is supposed to relieve tension and enhance energy flow when placed on the foot between the big toe and the second toe.

2. Spleen 6 (SP 6): Located in the inner thigh above the ankle, it is linked to digestive health and menstruation discomfort.

3. Kidney 1 (KD 1): Located near the bottom of the foot, it is said to link the body

to the energy of the earth, offering stability and anchoring.

Hand And Foot Points

1. Union Valley (LI 4): As previously stated, it is located between the thumb and index finger and is said to be effective for a variety of ailments, including tension headaches and pain alleviation.

2. Bigger Rushing (LV 3): It's said to help with stress relief since it's located on the top of the foot, between the first and second toes.

3. Inner Gate (PC 6): Located on the inner forearm, about three fingers' breadth from the wrist crease, it is believed to relieve nausea and motion sickness.

Understanding and activating these essential acupressure sites will help novices begin their path toward stress management, relaxation, and perhaps reducing a variety of discomforts.

CHAPTER 4

Benefits Of Acupressure

Acupressure, an ancient therapeutic practice based on traditional Chinese medicine, has several physical, mental, and emotional advantages. Pressure is applied to certain areas of the body to activate natural healing processes and restore equilibrium. The following are the several advantages:

Physical Health Benefits

Acupressure is well-known for its ability to treat a variety of physical illnesses and enhance overall wellness:

• **Pain Relief:** Acupressure may relieve pain from headaches, migraines, muscular strain, joint discomfort, and menstrual cramps by targeting particular pressure points. Endorphins, the body's natural painkillers, are released when these sites are stimulated.

• Improved Circulation: Applying pressure to meridian points improves blood circulation throughout the body, resulting in improved oxygen and nutrient distribution.

• Improved Immune System: Regular acupressure treatments may help to improve the immune system, possibly lowering disease frequency and improving the body's natural defensive systems.

• Digestive Health: Stimulating certain areas may help with digestion and relieve indigestion, bloating, and constipation problems.

Mental And Emotional Well-Being

Acupressure improves mental health by fostering relaxation and emotional balance:

• Tension Reduction: Applying pressure to certain spots helps relieve tension and anxiety, fostering calm and relaxation.

• Greater Sleep Quality: Acupressure may aid in the management of sleep problems by generating relaxation and relieving tension, resulting in greater sleep quality.

• Emotional Stability: Acupressure may help control emotions by balancing the flow of Qi, minimizing mood swings, and improving emotional stability.

Holistic Healing With Acupressure

Acupressure, in addition to treating particular ailments, represents a comprehensive approach to healing:

• Energy Flow Balancing: Acupressure strives to restore equilibrium inside the body by regulating the flow of energy (Qi) via meridians, treating the fundamental cause of imbalances.

• Self-awareness and Mindfulness: Acupressure commonly includes mindfulness methods, which promote self-awareness and improve the mind-body connection.

• **Preventative Care:** Regular acupressure treatments may be used to maintain general well-being and avoid the emergence of certain disorders.

With its many advantages, acupressure provides a natural and non-invasive technique to enhance health and well-being. It is critical to view acupressure as a complementary therapy to traditional medical treatments and to consult with a certified practitioner for assistance and individualized sessions.

This chapter introduces the transforming power of acupressure, showing its wide range of advantages for those seeking holistic treatment and better well-being.

CHAPTER 5

Acupressure For Common Ailments

Stress And Anxiety Relief

Acupressure is a natural and efficient way to relieve tension and anxiety. Applying pressure to certain places on the body relieves stress, promotes relaxation, and lowers cortisol levels. When stimulated regularly, points such as the Third Eye (Yintang), Inner Gate (Neiguan), and Heavenly Pillar (B10) are known to quiet the mind and ease tension. The technique promotes deep breathing, which aids in relaxation responses.

Pain Management

One of the amazing uses of acupressure is in the treatment of pain, such as headaches, menstrual cramps, back pain, and others. Acupressure stimulates endorphin release by targeting pressure points such as the Union Valley (LI4) for headaches or the Lower Back Shu (UB23) for back discomfort, alleviating pain and supporting natural healing processes. Regular sessions may help to alleviate chronic pain symptoms and boost general well-being.

Sleep Disorders And Insomnia

By resolving imbalances in the body's energy flow, acupressure may help improve sleep quality and cure insomnia.

Spirit Gate (HT7) and Inner Frontier Gate (P6) points are often activated to encourage relaxation and better sleep. When used before bedtime, acupressure methods promote tranquility, lowering restlessness and assisting folks in falling asleep more quickly.

Acupressure's holistic nature goes beyond symptom treatment. It seeks to restore equilibrium to the body's energy channels, hence improving general health. The practice tackles particular diseases while also boosting the body's self-healing capabilities, creating balance in physical, mental, and emotional components.

The mild but powerful effects of acupressure make it a diverse and accessible tool for treating common health difficulties, encouraging people to take control of their health via natural, non-invasive ways.

While acupressure may be very effective, it is critical to speak with a skilled practitioner before using it, particularly for chronic problems or in combination with other medical therapies.

CHAPTER 6

Incorporating Acupressure Into Daily Life

As a natural and accessible therapeutic approach, acupressure may be easily incorporated into everyday routines, providing several advantages for self-care, family, and general health practices.

Self-Care Practices

Understanding and applying acupressure methods may considerably improve one's well-being. Techniques including applying light pressure or massage to particular places on the body may reduce stress, increase relaxation, and boost overall vitality. This chapter goes into self-administered acupressure regimens, which allow people to manage stress, headaches, and exhaustion, and even improve digestion or sleep. Furthermore, experimenting with acupressure for stress release in the neck, shoulders, and back as a result of long hours of sitting or repeated chores may be quite effective.

Using Acupressure For Family And Friends

Learning acupressure methods enables you to share the advantages with family and friends. This section focuses on basic, safe, and efficient acupressure techniques for treating common discomforts such as headaches, stomach difficulties, and mild pains.

the fundamentals enables people to give assistance and support to family members or friends in need. For those who are unfamiliar with acupressure, it stresses the need for gentle procedures and correct direction.

Integrating Acupressure Into Wellness Routines

Including acupressure in wellness routines increases its efficacy. This section covers combining acupressure with other holistic activities such as meditation, yoga, or aromatherapy to provide a more holistic approach to health. Understanding how acupressure interacts with different wellness methods helps in the development of a balanced regimen that supports physical, mental, and emotional well-being.

Furthermore, it investigates the application of acupressure in certain health techniques, such as reflexology, traditional Chinese medicine, or energy work, to enhance its benefits. Individuals might be encouraged to investigate and benefit from a holistic approach to health by emphasizing the synergy between diverse therapeutic modalities.

This chapter seeks to provide novices with practical information and practices that will allow them to use acupressure as a valued and accessible tool in their everyday life, not only for instant relief but as an important part of their overall well-being plan.

CHAPTER 7

Safety And Precautions In Acupressure

When used appropriately, acupressure as an alternative medicine is typically safe. However, some safety precautions and procedures must be followed to guarantee a good and risk-free experience.

Understanding Limits And Boundaries

1. Self-awareness: It is critical to recognize personal boundaries and avoid using excessive force while performing acupressure. Overstimulation or applying too much pressure to certain spots may cause pain or harm.

2. **Pregnancy:** Some pressure points are not recommended during pregnancy because they may cause contractions or harm the baby. Before utilizing acupressure during pregnancy, it is best to consult with a certified healthcare expert.

3. **Children and the Elderly:** It is critical to use mild and lighter pressure when administering acupressure to children and the elderly to prevent pain or harm.

Special Considerations And Contradictions

1. **Medical Conditions:** People who have fractures, open wounds, severe osteoporosis, or cancer should exercise caution or avoid

using acupressure on affected regions without first contacting a healthcare expert.

2. People with chronic health difficulties, such as diabetes or cardiovascular disease, should consult their healthcare professional before using acupressure, particularly on sites that may influence these disorders.

3. Allergies and Skin Sensitivity: Some people may suffer from sensitive skin or allergies. It is best to use clean hands and avoid applying prolonged or excessive pressure to delicate skin regions.

When To Seek Professional Help

1. Persistent Symptoms: If symptoms continue or worsen after using acupressure, seek medical attention immediately.

2.   Unexplainable   discomfort   or Discomfort: If applying pressure to certain places produces acute or unexplainable discomfort, cease immediately and seek a healthcare expert.

3. Safety in Training and information: Acupressure may have unwanted adverse effects if applied poorly or without sufficient information. Seeking advice from skilled experts or licensed teachers is advantageous, particularly for beginners.

When practicing acupressure, safety is of the utmost importance. Understanding the body's reaction, understanding individual limits, and being aware of particular situations that may exclude acupressure are all necessary for a happy and safe experience. Always prioritize your health and seek expert advice when necessary.

CHAPTER 8

Combining Acupressure With Other Modalities

Acupressure, which has its roots in ancient Eastern healing methods, works well with a variety of modalities, enhancing therapeutic potential and overall well-being. Integrating acupressure with other therapeutic traditions may increase its efficacy and treat a broader range of health conditions.

Acupressure And Traditional Chinese Medicine (TCM)

Acupressure has its roots in Traditional Chinese Medicine and works in tandem with acupuncture, herbal medicine, and Qigong.

TCM promotes balance and harmony throughout the body's systems in its holistic approach to health. Acupressure effects are enhanced when combined with TCM concepts of meridians, qi flow, and yin-yang balance. Acupressure practitioners often mix it with herbal medicines or propose certain dietary changes to enhance its benefits.

Acupressure And Western Medicine

In recent years, there has been a growing acceptance of complementary treatments such as acupressure in combination with Western medicine. Several medical practitioners recognize its value in supplementing traditional therapy. Acupressure may be used as an additional treatment to help with pain alleviation, stress reduction, and mental wellness. Many hospitals and clinics use integrative treatments, such as acupressure, in addition to regular medical therapy to improve patient outcomes.

Complementary Therapies And Acupressure

Massage therapy, aromatherapy, reflexology, and yoga are all complementary treatments that work well with acupressure. When these techniques are integrated, they provide a complete approach to well-being, addressing diverse aspects of physical, emotional, and mental health. Combining acupressure with massage, for example, increases relaxation, relieves muscle tension, and boosts general vitality. Similarly, combining acupressure with yoga or meditation improves consciousness, which aids in stress reduction and emotional balance.

A Multidisciplinary Approach to Holistic Health

Acupressure combined with other therapeutic methods provides for a multidisciplinary approach to health and wellbeing. Such an approach recognizes that each person may react differently to therapies and that combining diverse ways may result in more complete outcomes. This all-encompassing approach seeks holistic well-being by taking into account the interdependence of mind, body, and spirit.

Practitioners working together

Collaboration among acupressure practitioners, Western medical experts, and other holistic healers promotes a complete healthcare network. Encouragement of communication and cooperation among practitioners allows for a more nuanced knowledge of patient needs, which leads to individualized treatment programs adapted to individual needs.

Integrating acupressure with other modalities broadens its potential, providing a broader range of therapeutic effects and enhancing overall wellness. Individuals may access a broad variety of resources to improve their well-being by adopting a collaborative approach and recognizing the synergy between varied therapeutic approaches.

CHAPTER 9

Advanced Acupressure Techniques

Acupressure Massage

Acupressure massage is applying pressure to certain places on the body to promote the body's inherent healing powers. Finger pressure, kneading, tapping, and moderate stretching are some of the techniques used. The goal is to relieve stress, increase circulation, and induce relaxation. Understanding the body's meridian points is critical for acupressure massage targeting the correct places. Depending on the condition being treated or the intended objective, such as easing muscular tension, lowering stress, or improving general well-being, several massage methods may be utilized.

Acupressure In Traditional Healing Systems

Acupressure is used in many traditional healing systems, including Traditional Chinese Medicine (TCM) and Ayurveda. Acupressure is a vital part of TCM that is used to balance the body's energy flow or Qi. To accomplish holistic healing, it is often paired with herbal medicines, dietary modifications, and other therapies. Ayurveda, an ancient Indian school of medicine, employs similar ideas, concentrating on energy balance and health improvement using acupressure-like treatments.

Exploring Acupressure Variations

Acupressure comes in many forms and variants, each with its emphasis and methodology. Jin Shin Jyutsu, which uses gentle touch on specific points to balance energy flows; Shiatsu, a Japanese form that involves applying pressure along meridians to improve overall well-being; and Reflexology, which focuses on pressure points in the feet, hands, and ears that correspond to specific organs and systems in the body. Exploring these differences may provide a variety of options for addressing specific health conditions or improving general well-being.

Understanding advanced acupressure methods may help to develop one's practice and increase one's range of possible treatments. Each method provides distinct insights into the body's energy systems and may be tailored to meet individual requirements, making acupressure a flexible and adaptable therapeutic practice for improving health and well-being.

CHAPTER 10

The Future Of Acupressure

Acupressure, an old therapeutic technique, is ever-evolving, using new science and increasing technology while remaining grounded in traditional methods. This chapter explores the future advancements and possibilities for acupressure.

Modern Research And Advancements

Technological advancements have allowed for a better understanding of the physiological mechanics behind acupressure. Functional MRI (magnetic resonance imaging) and other imaging methods are being used to investigate the neurological basis of acupressure's effects. Future studies may concentrate on improving these scientific experiments to better understand how activating acupoints affects the body's internal systems, ranging from the neurological and circulatory to the endocrine.

Furthermore, there is a rising interest in evidence-based medicine, which is encouraging further scientific research to evaluate the usefulness of acupressure in treating a variety of illnesses. This study may result in more defined methods and standards for the use of acupressure in hospital settings.

Evolving Trends In Acupressure

As interest in holistic treatment grows, acupressure is positioned to play a larger role. Integration into traditional medical treatments, as well as cooperation between acupressure practitioners and healthcare professionals, are expected. Acupressure may be used in pain clinics, maternity care, mental health institutions, and palliative care units in the future.

Technological advances may also result in new acupressure tools and gadgets. From wearable gadgets that stimulate particular acupoints to smartphone applications that guide self-administered acupressure, the future offers the promise of a more accessible and user-friendly approach to acupressure treatments.

The Role Of Acupressure In Holistic Healthcare

Acupressure as a supplementary treatment might be further integrated into holistic healthcare, which focuses on treating the full person—mind, body, and spirit. Acupressure may become a vital aspect of tailored wellness regimens due to its non-invasive nature and capacity to treat a broad variety of physical, emotional, and mental disorders.

Educational efforts and training programs for healthcare workers may raise knowledge and understanding of the advantages of acupressure, leading to better educated and holistic patient care.

Finally, with continued study, technology breakthroughs, and growing acceptance in integrative healthcare, the future of acupressure is positive. As the healthcare environment evolves, acupressure is projected to play an important role in promoting well-being and delivering holistic treatment to people all over the globe.

Conclusion

"We've embarked on a fascinating exploration of ancient healing techniques blended with modern understanding in this journey through the fundamentals of acupressure.

Acupressure, rooted in the philosophy of balancing life energies, reveals a world where simple pressure on specific points can foster wellness and vitality. We've delved into the foundational concepts of Qi, meridians, Yin-Yang balance, and the Five Elements theory, essential pillars of acupressure practice."

We've discovered the transformative power at our fingertips by learning about pressure points, tools, and techniques. Acupressure, a modality with numerous benefits, goes beyond simply relieving physical discomfort; it also helps to relieve mental stress, manage pain, and improve sleep quality.

Furthermore, as we've progressed, we've seen a more complex landscape of advanced treatments, such as specialized massage, and their incorporation into many traditional healing systems, emphasizing the depth and versatility of acupressure.

Looking forward, the future of acupressure is hopeful, with continuing study and breakthroughs constantly revealing its potential; as it advances, acupressure is set to play an important part in holistic healthcare, contributing to a more balanced and integrated approach to well-being.

Remember that this introduction just scrapes the surface of a large and sophisticated healing art; the investigation of acupressure is an ongoing journey that invites us to further comprehend, practice, and feel its great advantages, fostering harmony within ourselves and our environs.

THE END